DOCTORS VISITS TRACKER

Keep a Track of
Doctors Visits and Notes

This Tracker belongs to:

_____

DATE OF VISIT: _____

REASON FOR VISIT: _____

_____

PHYSICIAN/CLINIC: _____

QUESTIONS TO ASK: _____

_____

_____

_____

NOTES: _____

_____

_____

_____

_____

_____

_____

PRESCRIPTIONS: _____

_____

_____

NEXT APPOINTMENT: _____

DATE OF VISIT: _____

REASON FOR VISIT: _____

_____

PHYSICIAN/CLINIC: _____

QUESTIONS TO ASK: _____

_____

_____

_____

NOTES: _____

_____

_____

_____

_____

_____

_____

PRESCRIPTIONS: _____

_____

_____

NEXT APPOINTMENT: _____

DATE OF VISIT: _____

REASON FOR VISIT: _____

_____

PHYSICIAN/CLINIC: _____

QUESTIONS TO ASK: _____

_____

_____

_____

NOTES: _____

_____

_____

_____

_____

_____

_____

PRESCRIPTIONS: _____

_____

_____

NEXT APPOINTMENT: _____

DATE OF VISIT: _____

REASON FOR VISIT: _____

_____

PHYSICIAN/CLINIC: _____

QUESTIONS TO ASK: _____

_____

_____

_____

NOTES: _____

_____

_____

_____

_____

_____

_____

PRESCRIPTIONS: _____

_____

_____

NEXT APPOINTMENT: _____

DATE OF VISIT: _____

REASON FOR VISIT: _____

_____

PHYSICIAN/CLINIC: _____

QUESTIONS TO ASK: _____

_____

_____

_____

NOTES: _____

_____

_____

_____

_____

_____

_____

PRESCRIPTIONS: _____

_____

_____

NEXT APPOINTMENT: _____

DATE OF VISIT: _____

REASON FOR VISIT: _____

_____

PHYSICIAN/CLINIC: _____

QUESTIONS TO ASK: _____

_____

_____

_____

NOTES: _____

_____

_____

_____

_____

_____

PRESCRIPTIONS: _____

_____

_____

NEXT APPOINTMENT: _____

DATE OF VISIT: _____

REASON FOR VISIT: _____

_____

PHYSICIAN/CLINIC: _____

QUESTIONS TO ASK: _____

_____

_____

_____

NOTES: _____

_____

_____

_____

_____

_____

PRESCRIPTIONS: _____

_____

_____

NEXT APPOINTMENT: _____

DATE OF VISIT: _____

REASON FOR VISIT: _____

_____

PHYSICIAN/CLINIC: _____

QUESTIONS TO ASK: _____

_____

_____

_____

NOTES: _____

_____

_____

_____

_____

_____

_____

PRESCRIPTIONS: _____

_____

_____

NEXT APPOINTMENT: _____

DATE OF VISIT: _____

REASON FOR VISIT: _____

_____

PHYSICIAN/CLINIC: _____

QUESTIONS TO ASK: _____

_____

_____

_____

NOTES: _____

_____

_____

_____

_____

_____

PRESCRIPTIONS: _____

_____

_____

NEXT APPOINTMENT: _____

DATE OF VISIT: _____

REASON FOR VISIT: _____

_____

PHYSICIAN/CLINIC: _____

QUESTIONS TO ASK: _____

_____

_____

_____

NOTES: _____

_____

_____

_____

_____

_____

PRESCRIPTIONS: _____

_____

_____

NEXT APPOINTMENT: _____

DATE OF VISIT: _____

REASON FOR VISIT: _____

_____

PHYSICIAN/CLINIC: _____

QUESTIONS TO ASK: _____

_____

_____

_____

NOTES: _____

_____

_____

_____

_____

_____

_____

PRESCRIPTIONS: _____

_____

_____

NEXT APPOINTMENT: _____

DATE OF VISIT: _____

REASON FOR VISIT: _____

_____

PHYSICIAN/CLINIC: _____

QUESTIONS TO ASK: _____

_____

_____

_____

NOTES: _____

_____

_____

_____

_____

_____

_____

PRESCRIPTIONS: _____

_____

_____

NEXT APPOINTMENT: _____

DATE OF VISIT: _____

REASON FOR VISIT: _____

_____

PHYSICIAN/CLINIC: _____

QUESTIONS TO ASK: _____

_____

_____

_____

NOTES: _____

_____

_____

_____

_____

_____

_____

PRESCRIPTIONS: _____

_____

_____

NEXT APPOINTMENT: _____

DATE OF VISIT: _____

REASON FOR VISIT: _____

_____

PHYSICIAN/CLINIC: _____

QUESTIONS TO ASK: _____

_____

_____

_____

NOTES: _____

_____

_____

_____

_____

_____

_____

PRESCRIPTIONS: _____

_____

_____

NEXT APPOINTMENT: _____

DATE OF VISIT: _____

REASON FOR VISIT: _____

_____

PHYSICIAN/CLINIC: _____

QUESTIONS TO ASK: _____

_____

_____

_____

NOTES: _____

_____

_____

_____

_____

_____

PRESCRIPTIONS: _____

_____

_____

NEXT APPOINTMENT: _____

DATE OF VISIT: _____

REASON FOR VISIT: _____

_____

PHYSICIAN/CLINIC: _____

QUESTIONS TO ASK: _____

_____

_____

_____

NOTES: _____

_____

_____

_____

_____

_____

_____

PRESCRIPTIONS: _____

_____

_____

NEXT APPOINTMENT: _____

DATE OF VISIT: _____

REASON FOR VISIT: _____

_____

PHYSICIAN/CLINIC: _____

QUESTIONS TO ASK: _____

_____

_____

_____

NOTES: _____

_____

_____

_____

_____

_____

_____

PRESCRIPTIONS: _____

_____

_____

NEXT APPOINTMENT: _____

DATE OF VISIT: _____

REASON FOR VISIT: _____

_____

PHYSICIAN/CLINIC: _____

QUESTIONS TO ASK: _____

_____

_____

_____

NOTES: _____

_____

_____

_____

_____

_____

PRESCRIPTIONS: _____

_____

_____

NEXT APPOINTMENT: _____

DATE OF VISIT: _____

REASON FOR VISIT: _____

_____

PHYSICIAN/CLINIC: _____

QUESTIONS TO ASK: _____

_____

_____

_____

NOTES: _____

_____

_____

_____

_____

_____

_____

PRESCRIPTIONS: _____

_____

_____

NEXT APPOINTMENT: _____

DATE OF VISIT: _____

REASON FOR VISIT: _____

_____

PHYSICIAN/CLINIC: _____

QUESTIONS TO ASK: _____

_____

_____

_____

NOTES: _____

_____

_____

_____

_____

_____

_____

PRESCRIPTIONS: _____

_____

_____

NEXT APPOINTMENT: _____

DATE OF VISIT: _____

REASON FOR VISIT: _____

_____

PHYSICIAN/CLINIC: _____

QUESTIONS TO ASK: _____

_____

_____

_____

NOTES: _____

_____

_____

_____

_____

_____

PRESCRIPTIONS: _____

_____

_____

NEXT APPOINTMENT: _____

DATE OF VISIT: _____

REASON FOR VISIT: _____

_____

PHYSICIAN/CLINIC: _____

QUESTIONS TO ASK: _____

_____

_____

_____

NOTES: _____

_____

_____

_____

_____

_____

_____

PRESCRIPTIONS: _____

_____

_____

NEXT APPOINTMENT: _____

DATE OF VISIT: _____

REASON FOR VISIT: _____

_____

PHYSICIAN/CLINIC: _____

QUESTIONS TO ASK: _____

_____

_____

_____

NOTES: _____

_____

_____

_____

_____

_____

_____

PRESCRIPTIONS: _____

_____

_____

NEXT APPOINTMENT: _____

DATE OF VISIT: _____

REASON FOR VISIT: _____

_____

PHYSICIAN/CLINIC: _____

QUESTIONS TO ASK: _____

_____

_____

_____

NOTES: _____

_____

_____

_____

_____

_____

_____

PRESCRIPTIONS: _____

_____

_____

NEXT APPOINTMENT: _____

DATE OF VISIT: _____

REASON FOR VISIT: _____

_____

PHYSICIAN/CLINIC: _____

QUESTIONS TO ASK: _____

_____

_____

_____

NOTES: _____

_____

_____

_____

_____

_____

_____

PRESCRIPTIONS: _____

_____

_____

NEXT APPOINTMENT: _____

DATE OF VISIT: _____

REASON FOR VISIT: _____

_____

PHYSICIAN/CLINIC: _____

QUESTIONS TO ASK: _____

_____

_____

_____

NOTES: _____

_____

_____

_____

_____

_____

_____

PRESCRIPTIONS: _____

_____

_____

NEXT APPOINTMENT: _____

DATE OF VISIT: _____

REASON FOR VISIT: _____

_____

PHYSICIAN/CLINIC: _____

QUESTIONS TO ASK: _____

_____

_____

_____

NOTES: _____

_____

_____

_____

_____

_____

PRESCRIPTIONS: _____

_____

_____

NEXT APPOINTMENT: _____

DATE OF VISIT: _____

REASON FOR VISIT: _____

_____

PHYSICIAN/CLINIC: _____

QUESTIONS TO ASK: _____

_____

_____

_____

NOTES: _____

_____

_____

_____

_____

_____

_____

PRESCRIPTIONS: _____

_____

_____

NEXT APPOINTMENT: _____

DATE OF VISIT: _____

REASON FOR VISIT: _____

_____

PHYSICIAN/CLINIC: _____

QUESTIONS TO ASK: _____

_____

_____

_____

NOTES: _____

_____

_____

_____

_____

_____

PRESCRIPTIONS: _____

_____

_____

NEXT APPOINTMENT: _____

DATE OF VISIT: _____

REASON FOR VISIT: _____

_____

PHYSICIAN/CLINIC: _____

QUESTIONS TO ASK: _____

_____

_____

_____

NOTES: _____

_____

_____

_____

_____

_____

PRESCRIPTIONS: _____

_____

_____

NEXT APPOINTMENT: _____

DATE OF VISIT: _____

REASON FOR VISIT: _____

_____

PHYSICIAN/CLINIC: _____

QUESTIONS TO ASK: _____

_____

_____

_____

NOTES: _____

_____

_____

_____

_____

_____

_____

PRESCRIPTIONS: _____

_____

_____

NEXT APPOINTMENT: _____

DATE OF VISIT: _____

REASON FOR VISIT: _____

_____

PHYSICIAN/CLINIC: _____

QUESTIONS TO ASK: _____

_____

_____

_____

NOTES: _____

_____

_____

_____

_____

_____

_____

PRESCRIPTIONS: _____

_____

_____

NEXT APPOINTMENT: _____

DATE OF VISIT: _____

REASON FOR VISIT: _____

_____

PHYSICIAN/CLINIC: _____

QUESTIONS TO ASK: _____

_____

_____

_____

NOTES: _____

_____

_____

_____

_____

_____

_____

PRESCRIPTIONS: _____

_____

_____

NEXT APPOINTMENT: _____

DATE OF VISIT: _____

REASON FOR VISIT: _____

_____

PHYSICIAN/CLINIC: _____

QUESTIONS TO ASK: _____

_____

_____

_____

NOTES: _____

_____

_____

_____

_____

_____

_____

PRESCRIPTIONS: _____

_____

_____

NEXT APPOINTMENT: _____

DATE OF VISIT: _____

REASON FOR VISIT: _____

_____

PHYSICIAN/CLINIC: _____

QUESTIONS TO ASK: _____

_____

_____

_____

NOTES: _____

_____

_____

_____

_____

_____

_____

PRESCRIPTIONS: _____

_____

_____

NEXT APPOINTMENT: _____

DATE OF VISIT: _____

REASON FOR VISIT: _____

_____

PHYSICIAN/CLINIC: _____

QUESTIONS TO ASK: _____

_____

_____

_____

NOTES: _____

_____

_____

_____

_____

_____

_____

PRESCRIPTIONS: _____

_____

_____

NEXT APPOINTMENT: _____

DATE OF VISIT: _____

REASON FOR VISIT: _____

_____

PHYSICIAN/CLINIC: _____

QUESTIONS TO ASK: _____

_____

_____

_____

NOTES: _____

_____

_____

_____

_____

_____

_____

PRESCRIPTIONS: _____

_____

_____

NEXT APPOINTMENT: _____

DATE OF VISIT: _____

REASON FOR VISIT: _____

_____

PHYSICIAN/CLINIC: _____

QUESTIONS TO ASK: _____

_____

_____

_____

NOTES: _____

_____

_____

_____

_____

_____

_____

PRESCRIPTIONS: _____

_____

_____

NEXT APPOINTMENT: _____

DATE OF VISIT: _____

REASON FOR VISIT: _____

_____

PHYSICIAN/CLINIC: _____

QUESTIONS TO ASK: _____

_____

_____

_____

NOTES: _____

_____

_____

_____

_____

_____

PRESCRIPTIONS: _____

_____

_____

NEXT APPOINTMENT: _____

DATE OF VISIT: _____

REASON FOR VISIT: _____

_____

PHYSICIAN/CLINIC: _____

QUESTIONS TO ASK: _____

_____

_____

_____

NOTES: _____

_____

_____

_____

_____

_____

_____

PRESCRIPTIONS: _____

_____

_____

NEXT APPOINTMENT: _____

DATE OF VISIT: _____

REASON FOR VISIT: _____

_____

PHYSICIAN/CLINIC: _____

QUESTIONS TO ASK: _____

_____

_____

_____

NOTES: _____

_____

_____

_____

_____

_____

_____

PRESCRIPTIONS: _____

_____

_____

NEXT APPOINTMENT: _____

DATE OF VISIT: _____

REASON FOR VISIT: _____

_____

PHYSICIAN/CLINIC: _____

QUESTIONS TO ASK: _____

_____

_____

_____

NOTES: _____

_____

_____

_____

_____

_____

_____

PRESCRIPTIONS: _____

_____

_____

NEXT APPOINTMENT: _____

DATE OF VISIT: _____

REASON FOR VISIT: _____

_____

PHYSICIAN/CLINIC: _____

QUESTIONS TO ASK: _____

_____

_____

_____

NOTES: _____

_____

_____

_____

_____

_____

_____

PRESCRIPTIONS: _____

_____

_____

NEXT APPOINTMENT: _____

DATE OF VISIT: _____

REASON FOR VISIT: _____

_____

PHYSICIAN/CLINIC: _____

QUESTIONS TO ASK: _____

_____

_____

_____

NOTES: _____

_____

_____

_____

_____

_____

_____

PRESCRIPTIONS: _____

_____

_____

NEXT APPOINTMENT: _____

DATE OF VISIT: _____

REASON FOR VISIT: _____

_____

PHYSICIAN/CLINIC: _____

QUESTIONS TO ASK: _____

_____

_____

_____

NOTES: _____

_____

_____

_____

_____

_____

_____

PRESCRIPTIONS: _____

_____

_____

NEXT APPOINTMENT: _____

DATE OF VISIT: _____

REASON FOR VISIT: _____

_____

PHYSICIAN/CLINIC: _____

QUESTIONS TO ASK: _____

_____

_____

_____

NOTES: _____

_____

_____

_____

_____

_____

PRESCRIPTIONS: _____

_____

_____

NEXT APPOINTMENT: _____

DATE OF VISIT: _____

REASON FOR VISIT: _____

_____

PHYSICIAN/CLINIC: _____

QUESTIONS TO ASK: _____

_____

_____

_____

NOTES: _____

_____

_____

_____

_____

_____

PRESCRIPTIONS: _____

_____

_____

NEXT APPOINTMENT: _____

DATE OF VISIT: _____

REASON FOR VISIT: _____

_____

PHYSICIAN/CLINIC: _____

QUESTIONS TO ASK: _____

_____

_____

_____

NOTES: _____

_____

_____

_____

_____

_____

_____

PRESCRIPTIONS: _____

_____

_____

NEXT APPOINTMENT: _____

DATE OF VISIT: _____

REASON FOR VISIT: _____

_____

PHYSICIAN/CLINIC: _____

QUESTIONS TO ASK: _____

_____

_____

_____

NOTES: _____

_____

_____

_____

_____

_____

_____

PRESCRIPTIONS: _____

_____

_____

NEXT APPOINTMENT: _____

DATE OF VISIT: _____

REASON FOR VISIT: _____

_____

PHYSICIAN/CLINIC: _____

QUESTIONS TO ASK: _____

_____

_____

_____

NOTES: _____

_____

_____

_____

_____

_____

_____

PRESCRIPTIONS: _____

_____

_____

NEXT APPOINTMENT: _____

DATE OF VISIT: _____

REASON FOR VISIT: _____

_____

PHYSICIAN/CLINIC: _____

QUESTIONS TO ASK: _____

_____

_____

_____

NOTES: _____

_____

_____

_____

_____

_____

_____

PRESCRIPTIONS: _____

_____

_____

NEXT APPOINTMENT: _____

DATE OF VISIT: _____

REASON FOR VISIT: _____

_____

PHYSICIAN/CLINIC: _____

QUESTIONS TO ASK: _____

_____

_____

_____

NOTES: _____

_____

_____

_____

_____

_____

_____

PRESCRIPTIONS: _____

_____

_____

NEXT APPOINTMENT: _____

DATE OF VISIT: _____

REASON FOR VISIT: _____

_____

PHYSICIAN/CLINIC: _____

QUESTIONS TO ASK: _____

_____

_____

_____

NOTES: _____

_____

_____

_____

_____

_____

_____

PRESCRIPTIONS: _____

_____

_____

NEXT APPOINTMENT: _____

DATE OF VISIT: _____

REASON FOR VISIT: _____

_____

PHYSICIAN/CLINIC: _____

QUESTIONS TO ASK: _____

_____

_____

_____

NOTES: _____

_____

_____

_____

_____

_____

_____

PRESCRIPTIONS: _____

_____

_____

NEXT APPOINTMENT: _____

DATE OF VISIT: _____

REASON FOR VISIT: _____

_____

PHYSICIAN/CLINIC: _____

QUESTIONS TO ASK: _____

_____

_____

_____

NOTES: _____

_____

_____

_____

_____

_____

_____

PRESCRIPTIONS: _____

_____

_____

NEXT APPOINTMENT: _____

DATE OF VISIT: _____

REASON FOR VISIT: _____

_____

PHYSICIAN/CLINIC: _____

QUESTIONS TO ASK: _____

_____

_____

_____

NOTES: _____

_____

_____

_____

_____

_____

_____

PRESCRIPTIONS: _____

_____

_____

NEXT APPOINTMENT: _____

DATE OF VISIT: _____

REASON FOR VISIT: _____

_____

PHYSICIAN/CLINIC: _____

QUESTIONS TO ASK: _____

_____

_____

_____

NOTES: _____

_____

_____

_____

_____

_____

_____

PRESCRIPTIONS: _____

_____

_____

NEXT APPOINTMENT: _____

DATE OF VISIT: _____

REASON FOR VISIT: _____

_____

PHYSICIAN/CLINIC: _____

QUESTIONS TO ASK: _____

_____

_____

_____

NOTES: _____

_____

_____

_____

_____

_____

PRESCRIPTIONS: _____

_____

_____

NEXT APPOINTMENT: _____

DATE OF VISIT: _____

REASON FOR VISIT: _____

_____

PHYSICIAN/CLINIC: _____

QUESTIONS TO ASK: _____

_____

_____

_____

NOTES: _____

_____

_____

_____

_____

_____

PRESCRIPTIONS: _____

_____

_____

NEXT APPOINTMENT: _____

DATE OF VISIT: _____

REASON FOR VISIT: _____

_____

PHYSICIAN/CLINIC: _____

QUESTIONS TO ASK: _____

_____

_____

_____

NOTES: _____

_____

_____

_____

_____

_____

_____

PRESCRIPTIONS: _____

_____

_____

NEXT APPOINTMENT: _____

DATE OF VISIT: _____

REASON FOR VISIT: _____

_____

PHYSICIAN/CLINIC: _____

QUESTIONS TO ASK: _____

_____

_____

_____

NOTES: _____

_____

_____

_____

_____

_____

_____

PRESCRIPTIONS: _____

_____

_____

NEXT APPOINTMENT: _____

DATE OF VISIT: _____

REASON FOR VISIT: _____

_____

PHYSICIAN/CLINIC: _____

QUESTIONS TO ASK: _____

_____

_____

_____

NOTES: _____

_____

_____

_____

_____

_____

_____

PRESCRIPTIONS: _____

_____

_____

NEXT APPOINTMENT: _____

DATE OF VISIT: _____

REASON FOR VISIT: _____

_____

PHYSICIAN/CLINIC: _____

QUESTIONS TO ASK: _____

_____

_____

_____

NOTES: _____

_____

_____

_____

_____

_____

_____

PRESCRIPTIONS: _____

_____

_____

NEXT APPOINTMENT: _____

DATE OF VISIT: _____

REASON FOR VISIT: _____

_____

PHYSICIAN/CLINIC: _____

QUESTIONS TO ASK: _____

_____

_____

_____

NOTES: _____

_____

_____

_____

_____

_____

_____

PRESCRIPTIONS: _____

_____

_____

NEXT APPOINTMENT: _____

DATE OF VISIT: _____

REASON FOR VISIT: _____

_____

PHYSICIAN/CLINIC: _____

QUESTIONS TO ASK: _____

_____

_____

_____

NOTES: _____

_____

_____

_____

_____

_____

_____

PRESCRIPTIONS: _____

_____

_____

NEXT APPOINTMENT: _____

DATE OF VISIT: _____

REASON FOR VISIT: _____

_____

PHYSICIAN/CLINIC: _____

QUESTIONS TO ASK: _____

_____

_____

_____

NOTES: _____

_____

_____

_____

_____

_____

PRESCRIPTIONS: _____

_____

_____

NEXT APPOINTMENT: _____

DATE OF VISIT: _____

REASON FOR VISIT: _____

_____

PHYSICIAN/CLINIC: _____

QUESTIONS TO ASK: _____

_____

_____

_____

NOTES: _____

_____

_____

_____

_____

_____

PRESCRIPTIONS: _____

_____

_____

NEXT APPOINTMENT: _____

DATE OF VISIT: _____

REASON FOR VISIT: _____

_____

PHYSICIAN/CLINIC: _____

QUESTIONS TO ASK: _____

_____

_____

_____

NOTES: _____

_____

_____

_____

_____

_____

_____

PRESCRIPTIONS: _____

_____

_____

NEXT APPOINTMENT: _____

DATE OF VISIT: _____

REASON FOR VISIT: _____

_____

PHYSICIAN/CLINIC: _____

QUESTIONS TO ASK: _____

_____

_____

_____

NOTES: _____

_____

_____

_____

_____

_____

_____

PRESCRIPTIONS: _____

_____

_____

NEXT APPOINTMENT: _____

DATE OF VISIT: _____

REASON FOR VISIT: _____

_____

PHYSICIAN/CLINIC: _____

QUESTIONS TO ASK: _____

_____

_____

_____

NOTES: _____

_____

_____

_____

_____

_____

_____

PRESCRIPTIONS: _____

_____

_____

NEXT APPOINTMENT: _____

DATE OF VISIT: _____

REASON FOR VISIT: _____

_____

PHYSICIAN/CLINIC: _____

QUESTIONS TO ASK: _____

_____

_____

_____

NOTES: _____

_____

_____

_____

_____

_____

_____

PRESCRIPTIONS: _____

_____

_____

NEXT APPOINTMENT: _____

DATE OF VISIT: _____

REASON FOR VISIT: _____

_____

PHYSICIAN/CLINIC: _____

QUESTIONS TO ASK: _____

_____

_____

_____

NOTES: _____

_____

_____

_____

_____

_____

_____

PRESCRIPTIONS: _____

_____

_____

NEXT APPOINTMENT: _____

DATE OF VISIT: _____

REASON FOR VISIT: _____

_____

PHYSICIAN/CLINIC: _____

QUESTIONS TO ASK: _____

_____

_____

_____

NOTES: _____

_____

_____

_____

_____

_____

_____

PRESCRIPTIONS: _____

_____

_____

NEXT APPOINTMENT: _____

DATE OF VISIT: _____

REASON FOR VISIT: _____

_____

PHYSICIAN/CLINIC: _____

QUESTIONS TO ASK: _____

_____

_____

_____

NOTES: _____

_____

_____

_____

_____

_____

PRESCRIPTIONS: _____

_____

_____

NEXT APPOINTMENT: _____

DATE OF VISIT: _____

REASON FOR VISIT: _____

_____

PHYSICIAN/CLINIC: _____

QUESTIONS TO ASK: _____

_____

_____

_____

NOTES: _____

_____

_____

_____

_____

_____

_____

PRESCRIPTIONS: _____

_____

_____

NEXT APPOINTMENT: _____

DATE OF VISIT: _____

REASON FOR VISIT: _____

_____

PHYSICIAN/CLINIC: _____

QUESTIONS TO ASK: _____

_____

_____

_____

NOTES: _____

_____

_____

_____

_____

_____

_____

PRESCRIPTIONS: _____

_____

_____

NEXT APPOINTMENT: _____

DATE OF VISIT: _____

REASON FOR VISIT: _____

_____

PHYSICIAN/CLINIC: _____

QUESTIONS TO ASK: _____

_____

_____

_____

NOTES: _____

_____

_____

_____

_____

_____

_____

PRESCRIPTIONS: _____

_____

_____

NEXT APPOINTMENT: _____

DATE OF VISIT: _____

REASON FOR VISIT: _____

_____

PHYSICIAN/CLINIC: _____

QUESTIONS TO ASK: _____

_____

_____

_____

NOTES: _____

_____

_____

_____

_____

_____

_____

PRESCRIPTIONS: _____

_____

_____

NEXT APPOINTMENT: _____

DATE OF VISIT: _____

REASON FOR VISIT: _____

_____

PHYSICIAN/CLINIC: _____

QUESTIONS TO ASK: _____

_____

_____

_____

NOTES: _____

_____

_____

_____

_____

_____

_____

PRESCRIPTIONS: _____

_____

_____

NEXT APPOINTMENT: _____

DATE OF VISIT: _____

REASON FOR VISIT: _____

_____

PHYSICIAN/CLINIC: _____

QUESTIONS TO ASK: _____

_____

_____

_____

NOTES: _____

_____

_____

_____

_____

_____

_____

PRESCRIPTIONS: _____

_____

_____

NEXT APPOINTMENT: _____

DATE OF VISIT: _____

REASON FOR VISIT: _____

_____

PHYSICIAN/CLINIC: _____

QUESTIONS TO ASK: _____

_____

_____

_____

NOTES: _____

_____

_____

_____

_____

_____

_____

PRESCRIPTIONS: _____

_____

_____

NEXT APPOINTMENT: _____

DATE OF VISIT: _____

REASON FOR VISIT: _____

_____

PHYSICIAN/CLINIC: _____

QUESTIONS TO ASK: _____

_____

_____

_____

NOTES: _____

_____

_____

_____

_____

_____

_____

PRESCRIPTIONS: _____

_____

_____

NEXT APPOINTMENT: _____

DATE OF VISIT: _____

REASON FOR VISIT: _____

_____

PHYSICIAN/CLINIC: _____

QUESTIONS TO ASK: _____

_____

_____

_____

NOTES: _____

_____

_____

_____

_____

_____

_____

PRESCRIPTIONS: _____

_____

_____

NEXT APPOINTMENT: _____

DATE OF VISIT: _____

REASON FOR VISIT: _____

_____

PHYSICIAN/CLINIC: _____

QUESTIONS TO ASK: _____

_____

_____

_____

NOTES: _____

_____

_____

_____

_____

_____

_____

PRESCRIPTIONS: _____

_____

_____

NEXT APPOINTMENT: _____

DATE OF VISIT: _____

REASON FOR VISIT: _____

_____

PHYSICIAN/CLINIC: _____

QUESTIONS TO ASK: _____

_____

_____

_____

NOTES: _____

_____

_____

_____

_____

_____

_____

PRESCRIPTIONS: _____

_____

_____

NEXT APPOINTMENT: _____

DATE OF VISIT: _____

REASON FOR VISIT: _____

_____

PHYSICIAN/CLINIC: _____

QUESTIONS TO ASK: _____

_____

_____

_____

NOTES: _____

_____

_____

_____

_____

_____

_____

PRESCRIPTIONS: _____

_____

_____

NEXT APPOINTMENT: _____

DATE OF VISIT: _____

REASON FOR VISIT: _____

_____

PHYSICIAN/CLINIC: _____

QUESTIONS TO ASK: _____

_____

_____

_____

NOTES: _____

_____

_____

_____

_____

_____

PRESCRIPTIONS: _____

_____

_____

NEXT APPOINTMENT: _____

DATE OF VISIT: _____

REASON FOR VISIT: _____

_____

PHYSICIAN/CLINIC: _____

QUESTIONS TO ASK: _____

_____

_____

_____

NOTES: _____

_____

_____

_____

_____

_____

_____

PRESCRIPTIONS: _____

_____

_____

NEXT APPOINTMENT: _____

DATE OF VISIT: _____

REASON FOR VISIT: _____

_____

PHYSICIAN/CLINIC: _____

QUESTIONS TO ASK: _____

_____

_____

_____

NOTES: _____

_____

_____

_____

_____

_____

_____

PRESCRIPTIONS: _____

_____

_____

NEXT APPOINTMENT: _____

DATE OF VISIT: _____

REASON FOR VISIT: _____

_____

PHYSICIAN/CLINIC: _____

QUESTIONS TO ASK: _____

_____

_____

_____

NOTES: _____

_____

_____

_____

_____

_____

_____

PRESCRIPTIONS: _____

_____

_____

NEXT APPOINTMENT: _____

DATE OF VISIT: _____

REASON FOR VISIT: _____

_____

PHYSICIAN/CLINIC: _____

QUESTIONS TO ASK: _____

_____

_____

_____

NOTES: _____

_____

_____

_____

_____

_____

PRESCRIPTIONS: _____

_____

_____

NEXT APPOINTMENT: _____

DATE OF VISIT: _____

REASON FOR VISIT: _____

_____

PHYSICIAN/CLINIC: _____

QUESTIONS TO ASK: _____

_____

_____

_____

NOTES: _____

_____

_____

_____

_____

_____

_____

PRESCRIPTIONS: _____

_____

_____

NEXT APPOINTMENT: _____

DATE OF VISIT: _____

REASON FOR VISIT: _____

_____

PHYSICIAN/CLINIC: _____

QUESTIONS TO ASK: _____

_____

_____

_____

NOTES: _____

_____

_____

_____

_____

_____

PRESCRIPTIONS: _____

_____

_____

NEXT APPOINTMENT: _____

DATE OF VISIT: _____

REASON FOR VISIT: _____

_____

PHYSICIAN/CLINIC: _____

QUESTIONS TO ASK: _____

_____

_____

_____

NOTES: _____

_____

_____

_____

_____

_____

_____

PRESCRIPTIONS: _____

_____

_____

NEXT APPOINTMENT: _____

DATE OF VISIT: _____

REASON FOR VISIT: _____

_____

PHYSICIAN/CLINIC: _____

QUESTIONS TO ASK: _____

_____

_____

_____

NOTES: _____

_____

_____

_____

_____

_____

PRESCRIPTIONS: _____

_____

_____

NEXT APPOINTMENT: _____

DATE OF VISIT: _____

REASON FOR VISIT: _____

_____

PHYSICIAN/CLINIC: _____

QUESTIONS TO ASK: _____

_____

_____

_____

NOTES: _____

_____

_____

_____

_____

_____

_____

PRESCRIPTIONS: _____

_____

_____

NEXT APPOINTMENT: _____

DATE OF VISIT: _____

REASON FOR VISIT: _____

_____

PHYSICIAN/CLINIC: _____

QUESTIONS TO ASK: _____

_____

_____

_____

NOTES: _____

_____

_____

_____

_____

_____

_____

PRESCRIPTIONS: _____

_____

_____

NEXT APPOINTMENT: _____

DATE OF VISIT: _____

REASON FOR VISIT: _____

_____

PHYSICIAN/CLINIC: _____

QUESTIONS TO ASK: _____

_____

_____

_____

NOTES: _____

_____

_____

_____

_____

_____

_____

PRESCRIPTIONS: _____

_____

_____

NEXT APPOINTMENT: _____

DATE OF VISIT: _____

REASON FOR VISIT: _____

_____

PHYSICIAN/CLINIC: _____

QUESTIONS TO ASK: _____

_____

_____

_____

NOTES: _____

_____

_____

_____

_____

_____

PRESCRIPTIONS: _____

_____

_____

NEXT APPOINTMENT: _____

DATE OF VISIT: _____

REASON FOR VISIT: _____

_____

PHYSICIAN/CLINIC: _____

QUESTIONS TO ASK: _____

_____

_____

_____

NOTES: _____

_____

_____

_____

_____

_____

_____

PRESCRIPTIONS: _____

_____

_____

NEXT APPOINTMENT: _____

DATE OF VISIT: _____

REASON FOR VISIT: _____

_____

PHYSICIAN/CLINIC: _____

QUESTIONS TO ASK: _____

_____

_____

_____

NOTES: _____

_____

_____

_____

_____

_____

_____

PRESCRIPTIONS: _____

_____

_____

NEXT APPOINTMENT: _____

DATE OF VISIT: _____

REASON FOR VISIT: _____

_____

PHYSICIAN/CLINIC: _____

QUESTIONS TO ASK: _____

_____

_____

_____

NOTES: _____

_____

_____

_____

_____

_____

_____

PRESCRIPTIONS: _____

_____

_____

NEXT APPOINTMENT: _____

DATE OF VISIT: _____

REASON FOR VISIT: _____

_____

PHYSICIAN/CLINIC: _____

QUESTIONS TO ASK: _____

_____

_____

_____

NOTES: _____

_____

_____

_____

_____

_____

_____

PRESCRIPTIONS: _____

_____

_____

NEXT APPOINTMENT: _____

DATE OF VISIT: _____

REASON FOR VISIT: _____

_____

PHYSICIAN/CLINIC: _____

QUESTIONS TO ASK: _____

_____

_____

_____

NOTES: _____

_____

_____

_____

_____

_____

_____

PRESCRIPTIONS: _____

_____

_____

NEXT APPOINTMENT: _____

DATE OF VISIT: _____

REASON FOR VISIT: _____

_____

PHYSICIAN/CLINIC: _____

QUESTIONS TO ASK: _____

_____

_____

_____

NOTES: _____

_____

_____

_____

_____

_____

_____

PRESCRIPTIONS: _____

_____

_____

NEXT APPOINTMENT: _____

DATE OF VISIT: _____

REASON FOR VISIT: _____

_____

PHYSICIAN/CLINIC: _____

QUESTIONS TO ASK: _____

_____

_____

_____

NOTES: _____

_____

_____

_____

_____

_____

_____

PRESCRIPTIONS: _____

_____

_____

NEXT APPOINTMENT: _____

DATE OF VISIT: _____

REASON FOR VISIT: _____

_____

PHYSICIAN/CLINIC: _____

QUESTIONS TO ASK: _____

_____

_____

_____

NOTES: _____

_____

_____

_____

_____

_____

_____

PRESCRIPTIONS: _____

_____

_____

NEXT APPOINTMENT: _____

DATE OF VISIT: _____

REASON FOR VISIT: _____

_____

PHYSICIAN/CLINIC: _____

QUESTIONS TO ASK: _____

_____

_____

_____

NOTES: _____

_____

_____

_____

_____

_____

_____

PRESCRIPTIONS: _____

_____

_____

NEXT APPOINTMENT: _____

DATE OF VISIT: _____

REASON FOR VISIT: _____

_____

PHYSICIAN/CLINIC: _____

QUESTIONS TO ASK: _____

_____

_____

_____

NOTES: _____

_____

_____

_____

_____

_____

_____

PRESCRIPTIONS: _____

_____

_____

NEXT APPOINTMENT: _____

DATE OF VISIT: _____

REASON FOR VISIT: _____

_____

PHYSICIAN/CLINIC: _____

QUESTIONS TO ASK: _____

_____

_____

_____

NOTES: _____

_____

_____

_____

_____

_____

_____

PRESCRIPTIONS: _____

_____

_____

NEXT APPOINTMENT: _____

Made in the USA
Middletown, DE
03 August 2021